THE LONGEVITY CODE

THE LONGEVITY CODE

JULES HAWTHORNE

CONTENTS

1 Introduction   1
2 Chapter 1: Understanding Longevity   5
3 Chapter 2: Genetics and Longevity   7
4 Chapter 3: Lifestyle Choices and Longevity   9
5 Chapter 4: Mental Health and Longevity   13
6 Chapter 5: Emerging Technologies in Longevity Rese   17
7 Chapter 6: Longevity Across Cultures   21
8 Chapter 7: The Future of Longevity   25
9 Conclusion   27

Copyright © 2024 by Jules Hawthorne
All rights reserved. No part of this book may be reproduced in any manner whatsoever without written permission except in the case of brief quotations embodied in critical articles and reviews.
First Printing, 2024

CHAPTER 1

Introduction

Welcome to a revolution. Across the world and throughout history, millions of people have searched for a secret to a longer, healthier life. Humanity is now closer than ever to unlocking the key and solving the puzzle. Over the past century, human life expectancy has jumped from the mid-forties to about seventy-five years. Even more impressive is the substantial increase in life span of those past the mid-century mark. A woman aged fifty with few life-threatening diseases can now expect to live another thirty-three years: a fifty-year-old daughter can now expect to have a mother for more than an additional three decades. Throughout most of human history, life span has been limited to eighty to one hundred years. However, individuals are now clocking over one hundred years and those recently moving into their second century of life are the fastest growing segment of the population.

This demographic shift has clear implications for the health and longevity of our senior citizens and their family members as well as the caregiving demands on the workforce and broader economy. While most older adults age without chronic debilitating disease, one in two adults around the world suffers from one or more chronic conditions. According to the World Health Organization, chronic diseases such as cardiovascular disease, cancer, chronic lung disease, and diabetes are by far the leading cause of death worldwide—thirty-five million people die prematurely of a chronic condition every year. These diseases are responsible for two-thirds of deaths in the United States and account for 86 percent of America's health care costs.

The Significance of Longevity in Modern Society
Almost a third of Europeans over sixty-five are still in long-term relationships, and the habits of the mature tourist involve activities that now attract relatively few younger visitors. It's sobering to think that the word "retirement," with the idea of not working at all, didn't exist a century or so ago, because there were hardly any retirees to take advantage of it. Populations are aging everywhere, and this integration of older people into our everyday lives is causing rapid social change. It seems that everyone wants to grow old; no one wants to be old. Fifty-year-olds don't consider themselves old, but they begin to do so at seventy.

We live in the time of a great paradigm shift. In the developed world, as a result of the enormous strides made over the past century, violent death has all but disappeared from everyday experience. Life expectancy at the beginning of the twentieth century was just forty-nine years, so it is particularly remarkable that we have virtually doubled the normal human life span. But life span differs from life expectancy. Throughout human history, existing populations have included a few elderly survivors, a number of adults in the prime of life, and a great many children. As deaths in early life have become less common, populations have accumulated a greater number of middle-aged and elderly members. The increase in the number of older people in the population is occurring so quickly that we are having to redefine old age.

Purpose and Scope of the Book

The book is probably unique, as I have yet to find an equivalent. It is not written for the general public but those who are trying to make a change in their lifestyle. Those who have been poorly informed or have received conflicting or inconsistent messages and have at their disposal the means and opportunities to make changes but require evidence and a science-based approach. Nowadays, people are constantly bombarded with misinformation on many subjects, including longevity. The current status of the media complex is just to influence through a marketing approach. This is not how science is practiced! Reliability in the message is simply gone!

If you look up longevity on Amazon, you will find scores of books that have been written on the subject from every point of view. Thus, it is only fair to ask why yet another book on longevity, especially this one? Let me tell you upfront, I wrote this book to demonstrate that there is powerful science behind improving lifespan, and the sooner people learn about it, the better. It was written as a didactic tool for the public. The book does not require a background in medicine or science and is accessible to the public at large. Simplifying is a challenging task, because it requires a deep understanding and acquisition of the subject matter. It took me some time to write this book because it was an iterative learning curve over five years. You have the benefit of the final product.

CHAPTER 2

Chapter 1: Understanding Longevity

Every objective of growing up, finding a partner, and creating a family will be modified as we live on. Careers and education will undergo dramatic change in the face of lives lasting eighty or ninety or even more. Retirement, as we now think of it, is already a woefully outdated concept. Networks of support spanning multiple generations will become essential anchors, as parents, children, and sometimes grandchildren work together. Super longevity, the effects of medical technology and genetic engineering, is an impending and inevitable reality. That will be an even greater experience, indiscriminately embracing the wonder and heartbreak of extreme longevity. If we will all someday be living into our 90s, some researchers think it's possible to make 100 the functional maximum for humans. Our ability to stay vital and vigorous in those extra decades is the final race ahead of us.

To begin our journey, we must define the concept of longevity itself. It is quickly becoming more attractive as rapidly increasing life spans place new pressures on society and invoke the impulse for change in us individually. For the first time, the impacts of individual longevity are having a far-reaching snowball effect. It is no longer just the experts and philosophers contemplating the great social, economic, and lifestyle implications of these changes for the future.

Defining Longevity and Lifespan

Life expectancy has increased for different races and both sexes but not at the same pace. The interesting thing about the distribution of death is that it's not a sloping curve. In the United States, more and more people are living longer and longer. The number of women living to the age of one hundred is also increasing. While lifespan typically refers to how long a person has already lived, the phrase maximum lifespan more accurately conveys the concept of the upper limit of human existence. Maximum lifespan is the oldest any member of a group lives. For humans, the maximum lifespan has not changed appreciably. While the average American lifespan has increased nearly thirty years due to medical and technological changes, the maximum lifespan remains about 120 years. Although in some ways it may seem obtuse to distinguish between these terms—after all, a longer life is a longer life, right?—it's important to differentiate between the two when thinking about messages in the field. With extending longevity, we're pushing the average. To consider extending the maximum lifespan is asking much more of the task.

In setting up this book, let's make some definitions. First, let's distinguish the concepts of longevity and lifespan. Longevity refers to having a long life. Typically, it refers to how many years a person has lived. Statistics from the U.S. National Center for Health Statistics show that more and more people are enjoying longevity. In the United States, life expectancy at birth has increased from approximately fifty years around the time of the Civil War to about seventy-three years at the start of the twentieth century to nearly seventy-eight years today.

CHAPTER 3

Chapter 2: Genetics and Longevity

The net result of all of these processes is that most genes in the human genome typically exist in a few different flavors, or "alleles." Genes that celebrate this kind of flexibility are often said to be "polymorphic." Many polymorphisms, in turn, can subtly change the behavior of a protein or a gene, and hence, can have a very real impact on the body of the individual in question. If, among 1,000 people, one person has a rare allele in a gene that makes her one percent more likely to get to live a hundred years, and she actually makes it, arguably, that allele has "increased human longevity."

If you want to sculpt a new you out of hard work and exercise, it will help if you have the right genetic gifts for the body type you want to achieve. In the same way, if you want to push your body's "longevity genes," it will help if you understand what tools you're working with - how big is the club and how long is the fuse? Each of us has received two copies of each gene from each of our parents, so it's possible to possess two really healthy versions of a gene. On the other hand, (environmental and random mutations aside for the moment) it's possible to possess two copies of a gene that don't work very well. In the vast majority of cases though, the situation for any particular gene is not so clear-cut. From two different parents, an individual can end up with almost any combination of genetic variation, as a result of so-called "recombination" events that occur constantly on the chromosomes.

Genetic Factors Influencing Longevity

Nearly all the factors that influence successful aging are, to a greater or lesser extent, determined by our genetic inheritance. Although genes play only a part in influencing what we are like, this part goes some way towards determining health and wellbeing in old age.

Perhaps you have often wondered why some people live healthy and active lives into their late eighties or nineties while others become frail and bedridden in their sixties or seventies? The truth is that we do not know all the factors that determine why some people age so much better than others. However, we do know that a healthy life depends on a number of factors, including genetics, the environment, diet, and lifestyle. This is why there is so much opportunity for the application of new scientific discoveries in the field of aging and genetics. The experts will help you understand some of the scientific factors that influence healthy aging in this chapter so you can learn what steps you can take to promote a healthy, successful, longer life.

CHAPTER 4

Chapter 3: Lifestyle Choices and Longevity

You shouldn't be frustrated with information and advice we have all been given before. This is a cutting-edge book. It comes out of work at a research hub that has a mission of accelerating progress in the foundations of the life sciences. According to Dr. Steele, longevity is our 'next big challenge', and aging may be able to be treated as a disease because it is the biggest risk factor for many other diseases, and we're learning all the time about the molecular and cellular processes at work in our body. He includes in the book the personal story of his father's illness, but despite that personal hook, he has also given us other personal motivations. Not only is long life interesting, attainable or not, but he had always had a fascination with the concept and its portrayal in films and science fiction stories since childhood. So, in high school, he expected to work in the field after he studied his initial love, physics, but then realized a 'pretty much universal' error that other schools of biology were making.

In order to live a longer, healthier life, should we self-monitor our bodies as closely as some people monitor their stock portfolios? Andrew Steele thinks we might, and his book, The Longevity Code, aims to make the knowledge of those who do this accessible to the rest of us. One of his other premises is that we may not truly desire long life, despite our societal obsession with longevity, so we are forgoing information about it. Even if millions are tuning out when told about things they could do to lessen the burden of age-related diseases, for better or worse, he steeps you in some of the latest scientific research. Nutrients, enzymes, proteins: they fill the pages and our bodies. This is the journey Andrew Steele takes us on as we learn about the rules that govern the building of our cells, the DNA processes at work, and the information that together makes the intelligent system called our body.

Diet and Nutrition

Don Matesz, the author of Lanie's first book, has made significant improvements in the revised edition of the book, published after a thorough description of the Okinawa diet. He recommends that humans use foods that were consumed by Paleolithic humans, the hunters and gatherers, for most of human history, and provides scientific reasons for this. However, F.W. Potts found that Paleolithic humans had an intensive plant-based diet. Their health security, as well as that of the aforementioned Okinawans, should have been protected by food selections adapted to the genetic types of the people living on their respective main diets. However, in areas where the diet differs from genetic adaptation, such as the USA, some people, 80% of whom have serious degenerative and life-threatening diseases in their older years, may be protected by changes in diet that do not deviate from genetic restrictions. These dietary improvements are relatively recent compared to their genetic background, and genetic factors play a dominant role.

Different societies of the world consume a plant-based diet, calorie restriction, and/or fish. Eskimos, who live on fish and flesh food, are protected against arteriosclerosis and coronary diseases and live long lives. Okinawans, on the other hand, live over 100 years, with many living over 110 years, by eating a plant-based diet that is adapted to their genetic type. The main purpose of this book is to prevent or delay such diseases through adequate nutrients. Other books mention known means of aging retardation, but the writer has selected those for which nutritional means are known. A common idea is to rely on future high-tech and pharmaceutical means, but a Japanese article suggests that inexpensive nutritional methods must be found for the health security of aged people in less wealthy societies.

Physical Activity and Exercise

It is generally agreed that any amount of physical activity is better than nothing. Most recommendations suggest moderate-intensity aerobic exercise for at least 150 minutes per week for adults. These are physical activities that increase your heart rate and breathing and generally make you sweat for at least 10 minutes at a time. If you already meet these guidelines, you can focus on more vigorous activities or longer periods of them. Over time, try to integrate more at least twice a week in activities that work your major muscles like your legs, hips, back, abdomen, chest, shoulders, and arms. These activities increase muscle resistance by exercising weights, rubber bands, or your body's weight. Activities combining these approaches are highly recommended.

Unlike calorie consumption, humans exhibit a significant amount of individual variability in the amount of physical activity they engage in during their lives. When it comes to recommending physical activity, there is one piece of advice that stands out - exercise more. Virtually every clinical study on the subject has shown that there is a clear dose-response relationship between physical activity and improved health. In other words, the more active you are, the healthier you can become. There is general agreement that increased physical activity can reduce the risk of numerous age-related diseases.

CHAPTER 5

Chapter 4: Mental Health and Longevity

Late-life depression is not just a psychological state, but a severe, chronic disorder that is often part of a decline into decreasing health. In aging research, sugar is no longer seen as an energy source for muscles and organs, but as a major reason why the elderly suffer higher rates of type 2 diabetes, cognitive decline, high blood pressure, heart disease, and dental problems. Sugar can also make you appear older and be about ready to give up on life even before you reach 55.

After almost two decades researching how we age, I have come to believe that the concept of self isn't a very helpful guide to understanding aging. Individuals exist, but they are greatly influenced by their surroundings, and their physical and mental health and life expectancy are largely set by forces outside their brains. Whether you come from a large family with close relationships or a small or nonexistent relationship with a parent, your human DNA guides the communication between those cells and your immune system, digestion, and the process of repairing DNA through your entire life. Your vulnerability to everything from PTSD to schizophrenia can be determined by what your grandmother ate while pregnant.

Cognitive Function and Aging

The features of aging are influenced by sociocultural involvement, as shown by studies related to changes in personality and cognitive aging progress, studies conducted on semiotic interaction, and studies about the emotional environment in which human aging takes place. In order to keep cognitive health and memory strong, it is important to maintain mental and social stimulation. Being socially engaged, lifelong learning, and being physically and mentally active can help improve cognitive function. Other healthy habits, like physical exercise and healthy eating, can help reduce the risk of other chronic diseases, including certain types of dementia. These healthy habits are not only important for their own benefits, but they can be good for your overall health. In this age, physical exercise is beneficial for memory by stimulating the construction of specific regions of the cerebrum. The aging stage presents two features related to physical exercise: the execution of activities in high or moderate intensity. After intense physical exercise, older people succeed better in memorizing a specific task compared to people who did not run or ran with easy muscular effort, so as to breathe normally.

Cognitive health is an important part of successful aging. Intellectual aging is an interesting aspect of human aging. It consists of a process: it has no single list of properties. Many factors regulate this phenomenon, whether psychological or physiological in nature, or emerging after aging has appeared. In human aging, we note an increase in time latency and occasional forgetting incidents. Therefore, these phenomena lead to a decrease in the specificity of signals generated by cognitive function. For intellectual aging, among the psychological factors, important consequences for age organizations are evident: the decrease of attention skills, including the reaction speed to certain stimuli, the loss of the ability to memorize necessary data in unusual tasks, deficits regarding working memory, and the altered decision-making process. Among the physiological factors, increased time latency has priority, as well as forgetting incidents.

CHAPTER 6

Chapter 5: Emerging Technologies in Longevity Rese

Given that the basic principles of aging will be the same in humans as they are in other broadly similar organisms such as fruit flies, yeast, and worms, and given the short life span of many of these "lower" creatures and the many different ways that scientists could tinker with them to test their theories, you would be right to expect that the human genetic code would by now be giving up its secrets to allow us to pull the levers, plug the gaps, and so increase the human maximum life span and stave off age-related disease. Unfortunately, after three decades of delving into animal and human genetics, the story is not quite so encouraging. High modularity coupled with the simple and high aggregation of the molecular building blocks of life suggests a high degree of developmental and perhaps evolutionary constraint on the sequence of events that lead to high information content.

Genetics undoubtedly plays a significant role in the aging process. But why do some twins die young and others still go to yoga class at ninety? Why do some individuals live to be over one hundred? Many scientists reason that at least a good part of the answer may be found in how the fundamental blueprint provided by our genes is executed—a set of rules known as the genetic code. This genetic code is so deeply embedded in every part of the chemistry of the body and its response to the environment that it affects not only aging but also susceptibility to disease throughout our lives. In short, our genes tell us when to be born, when to grow, when to reproduce, and when to die. This raises a tantalizing question. Do these instructions create a timetable that is carved in stone by our genetic code, or do the genes play a more interactive role—a series of trade-offs that balance life, reproduction, and survival according to environmental conditions?

Advancements in Anti-Aging Therapies

In recent years, the search for anti-aging drugs has benefited from serendipity and from basic research in ways that suggest that remarkably powerful answers are now emerging. We have found previously unknown molecular targets for these drugs and discovered new ways to attack them. Radical new approaches that replace or rejuvenate worn-out organs are clearing the regulatory mists and entering the drug-development pipeline. The current health crisis that is caused by our rapidly aging population—the aging Armageddon—demands that these groundbreaking new therapies be perfected and applied to those in greatest need: people over sixty, who are at risk of dying from aging-related diseases. To date, physician-prescribed hormone replacements have constituted the most successful gerontological therapies, gradually putting off aging for a few additional years. Recently, an explosive series of discoveries that have eclipsed these hormone replacements have emerged disclose the decade-old approach of fixing aging at the root cause, to restore the function of organs made old by aging processes. These discoveries offer improvements in health that do not seem to have any side effects. The pace of these medical advances, already quite fast, is likely to grow even faster due to acceleration by the biotechnological gold-rush engine.

Most scientific research into human aging has been rooted in the concept of anti-aging drugs that can manipulate basic aging processes to keep organisms not just living longer but also remaining healthier. In years, this research has alternated between phases of pessimistic quiet, when science appeared to have given up trying to extend human lifespan, and periods of explosive epiphany, when a stream of powerful new life-extending discoveries gave pause to pessimism. We now seem to be awakening from the quiet period, with a stunning array of new biotechnological weapons that can not only increase healthspan—the period of life spent free of the diseases of aging—but also delay the onset of those diseases, thus increasing lifespan itself.

CHAPTER 7

Chapter 6: Longevity Across Cultures

Advertising has changed from "no cholesterol" to "low fat," to "low carbohydrate," to "low calorie," and now we have the fad diet of the month. As time has gone by, each fad diet has received more negative and harmful response. The word "hara-hachi-bunme" is a Japanese term used in Okinawa and means eat until you are 80% full. The term "little excess" is a general term that describes many cultures' belief in eating just a little less and avoiding getting full. The conclusion is that using different theories and different words and achieving better health is real. There is something Americans could use today: a 10% reduction in the number of obese people would save 8-11 million lives. This can happen because low carbohydrate diets have become extremely popular. In the future, the nation could very well experience a reduction in obesity levels. Until all the hoopla about low-carb is proven or disproven, the trade-in of extra carbs from the diet will result in reduced calories and a healthier ratio of carbohydrates to fats that will, maintained over time, lead to weight loss. The unique fact is that in order to survive, society has had to spend billions of dollars to keep its population from overindulging.

Okinawa, the Japanese island, was an agricultural community with a primarily rice-based agrarian economy. The Okinawan people were primarily followers of Buddhism. Generally, they did not overeat, and the average caloric intake was 1800 to 1900 calories per day. When a male Okinawan farmer reached the age of twenty and consumed an average of 270 or more calories from sugar, equivalent to a standard soft drink, he was asked by others if he was ill. As of this date, I have never seen a picture or drawing of an obese Okinawan farmer. In the early 1950s, the American government conducted an intensive study of the Japanese people. The study found that the diet of the Okinawans was equal to or greater than 85% plant-based caloric intake.

Comparative Studies on Longevity
These observations have encouraged scientists to investigate the dietary components which could account for this protection. Some dietary factors have been recognized to cause the majority of deaths in Western societies. Reducing the frequency of exposure to excessive alcohol and tobacco consumption has saved far more lives than any other public health measure. If excessive food intake and undernutrition are added to this list, a comprehensive public health policy would emerge. Despite all the pitfalls, the study of the lifestyle and genetic background of long-lived families is the most direct approach that we have to analyzing the interaction between environmental and genetic factors. The wealth of information accumulated in recent years by clinical, epidemiological, anthropological, biochemical, and biomedical research on dietary effects and disease as causes of accident has often failed to save lives, particularly those of the young. Animal experimentation has greatly expanded our knowledge of the mode of action of different dietary components.

Can the study of the mortality and morbidity of long-lived people complete the information?

The number of studies examining the eating habits of people who live to a ripe old age is staggering. This interest is justified by the observation that in most developed countries, the prevalence of the diseases associated with aging, particularly coronary heart disease, cancer, diabetes, and obesity, are lower in the aged. The example par excellence is the low prevalence of myocardial infarction (M.I.), stroke, and other manifestations of atherosclerosis observed in the elderly inhabitants (median age 85 years) of the Yugoslavian island of Korcula, collected between 1963 and 1978. In spite of consuming a high-fat diet, the incidence of arterial disease was similar to that of American men only of normal weight. A study of the nutritional habits of the Sardinian population, in which the men enjoy the same therapeutic value as those of the island of Korcula, revealed that the prevalence of diseases such as stomach cancer and breast cancer, which affect many young women, is much lower in the elderly. However, a causal link between this protection and nutrition has yet to be established.

CHAPTER 8

Chapter 7: The Future of Longevity

But for the millions of young people who currently are facing a future of abbreviated functional life, the future of longevity has profound importance. Their vision of a future filled with life should also be ours as a society. Indeed, success in fighting the war on aging and in developing rejuvenation strategies should be our national and global top priority. Currently, that isn't happening, but education will surely lead to proper prioritization.

The future of longevity looks very exciting to me. One could argue that having gotten you this far, you will join those who won't need to worry about the future of longevity. And you may well be right. Certainly, for people who are currently in good health and are enjoying an active lifestyle pursuing all of the things that make life fun, the addition of a few years or even a few decades may not seem of such great importance. In any event, your focus should be winning and maintaining great health. The rest comes along with that.

Predictions and Challenges in Longevity Science

Barring destructive accidents or unforeseen global disasters, extended longevity is a certainty for hominid evolution. Three major factors confirm the certainty. Evolutionary developmental clocks that do not expand the upper limit of the species' lifespan. The influence of slow life history speed on developing an extended human lifespan. Once a superlongevity age accessible to all is reached, humans may wish to stop aging and eliminate the duration of suffering among humans. Townes has emphasized the size and diversity of caring communities as an essential motivational factor in human evolution. He argues that the ongoing evolution of pro-social behaviors, such as altruism, has led to the expansion of concerns to at least some members of other species, and that such concerns have removed some of our most hurtful behaviors from our behavioral repertoire.

When it comes to the future of extreme longevity, I hesitate to make strong predictions. Predictions are difficult because the future is the product of random events and planned actions. That said, the future is forged through choices we make or neglect, and our choices may increase, decrease, or neutralize the benefits of extended lives. What follows is my best guess based on available evidence and the current state of scientific knowledge.

CHAPTER 9

Conclusion

The pace of development in biologic matters will set this book very clearly as a historical document. Such is the bewildering new world we inhabit. Some will be timeless, that is the implication that lifestyle is fundamentally responsible for our future health and longevity. To that extent, broadbrush statements should hold true for ways of maximizing the genetic inheritance you have, including such buried assumptions as positive attitude, nourishing social networks, having purpose throughout life and minimizing crises and losses will certainly maximize gene-powered benefits. We may not control our bodily hardware, but we do control the software. We can maximize our potential to stay younger longer. If this aids the quest of future, even more powerful interesting interventions into aging, then all the better. With luck, you will have dodged the bullet, for a while.

This is a book about aging, specifically how we as individuals can age more healthily and live for longer. It is an incredibly important topic simply because the worldwide population is old with a capital O. In the smoke-and-mirror world of genomics, where news can fade as fast as it arrives, we have been constantly reminded of a vision of ourselves as victims of our genes. The pace of contemporary understanding is phenomenal, but the promises offered can seem to be overplayed. It is, as we will see, one of the key themes in receiving, interpreting information about health from DNA. I hope to have cooked up a blend of key science and helpful, practical wisdom in combining the most up-to-date knowledge of human genetics with all current matters of obtaining a healthier life, generally dispensed with uncommon good sense. I say generally, in the knowledge that by writing at such a complex junction, my advice is essentially meted out as it stands today.

Key Takeaways and Actionable Steps

As we finish discussing all the elements of how to lead a longer, healthier life, it's time to summarize what we've learned throughout the book into key action steps. The primary goal of the book is to provide you with access to the appropriate tools and knowledge base you need in order to take control of your own health and life. Take the data and use it as you see fit to create and change the direction and outcome of your personal longevity roadmap. Unlike the countless types of diets you've heard about throughout your life (low carb, low fat, low protein, low calorie, fasting, time-dependent feeding, and meal skipping), our strategy does not focus on what goes into your mouth. Instead, we concentrate on quality, harmony, diversity, and restabilization. I call my plan, "The New-Stein Anti-die-t," because we're going to focus on the things that help keep you both alive and well.

Key Takeaways:

The U.S. healthcare system exists not as a system of health, but as a system of illness and its costly management. Healthcare needs to focus on the causes of poor health, not on disease treatment. Nutrition, exercise, sleep and lifestyle management are misunderstood and neglected in the practice of medicine, the policy of public health, and the attention of the patients. We need to equalize the nation's mission to perform sophisticated surgery. By ignoring these factors, America is leading the way in creating a nation not of prosperity and health, but of poverty and ill health. Why are we taking these medicines, drugs, and strange therapies? The use of our healthcare costs about $8,000 per year, depending on the data source. However, our healthcare ranking remains at 18th worldwide, in the United States. The quality and value that the "Founding Fathers" intended for the nation's inhabitants appears to be missing. Therefore, it becomes more and more crucial to our health and longevity to truly understand how our bodies handle food, physical activity, sleep, and lifestyle, and how we interact with the DNA and microbiome that affects our health. And then, based on that information, coach our biology to operate in the quest for better, healthier lives. Our health is ultimately in our hands and the information presented is all that allows the reader to begin their journey.

www.ingramcontent.com/pod-product-compliance
Lightning Source LLC
LaVergne TN
LVHW092102060526
838201LV00047B/1527